Keto Diet Recipes for Beginners

Breakfast Lunch Dinner

The Simple Keto Cookbook for Weight Loss. How to Create Quick and Easy Recipes in Less Than 30 Min, and Always be Fit Without Feeling on a Diet

Amy Newton

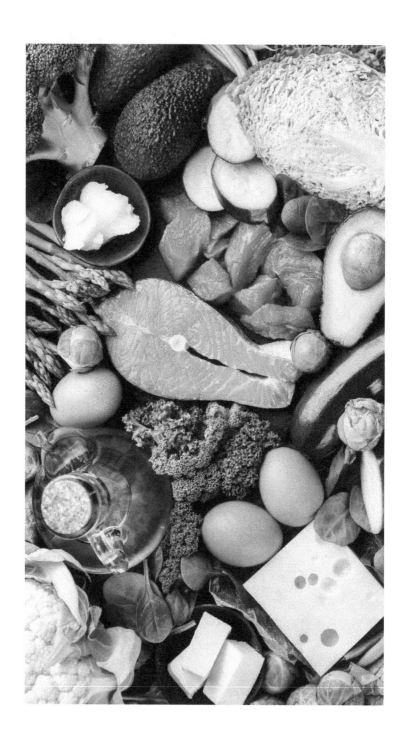

Table of Contents

Breakfast Recipes

1 French Omelet

Preparation Time: 10 minutes

Cooking Time: 10 minutes

Servings: 2

Ingredients:

2 large eggs

4 egg whites

¼ cup of milk

1/8 tsp of pepper

1/8 tsp of salt

1 cup of ham (cooked)

1 tbsp of green pepper (chopped)

1 tbsp of onion (chopped)

1/2 cup of cheddar cheese (shredded)

Directions

Whisk the first five listed ingredients.

Use a cooking spray for greasing a skillet. Place the skillet over medium flame. Add the mixture of eggs.

Cook for two minutes.

Top with the remaining ingredients. Fold the egg in half.

Cut the omelet in half. Serve immediately.

Nutrition: Calories: 189; Protein: 22.3 g; Carbs: 3.6 g; Fat: 10.9 g; Fiber: 0.1 g

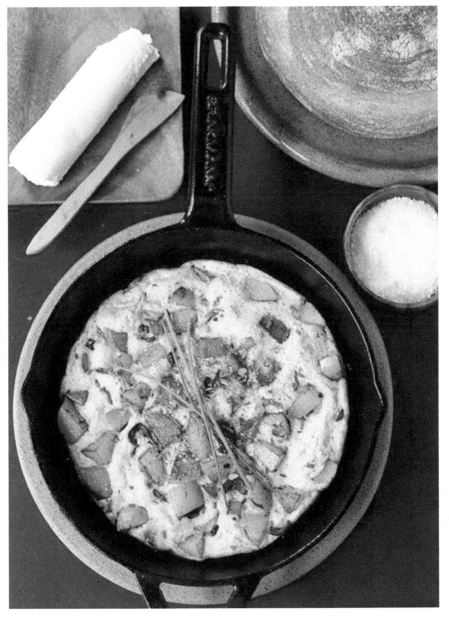

2 Sage Sausage Patty

Preparation Time: 10 minutes

Cooking Time: 10 hours 10 minutes

Servings: 8

Ingredients:

1 lb pork (ground)

3/4 cup cheddar cheese (ground)

1/4 cup buttermilk

1 tbsp onion (chopped)

2 tsp sage

3/4 tsp pepper

3/4 tsp salt

½ tsp oregano (dried)

½ tsp garlic powder

Directions:

Combine the listed ingredients either in a bowl or in a food processor.

Shape the mixture into eight equal patties of half-inch thickness. Refrigerate the patties for one hour.

Heat oil in an iron skillet. Cook the patties on each side for six minutes.

Serve hot.

Nutrition: Calories: 160.3; Protein: 14.6 g; Carbs: 1.2 g; Fat: 12.3 g; Fiber: 0.3 g

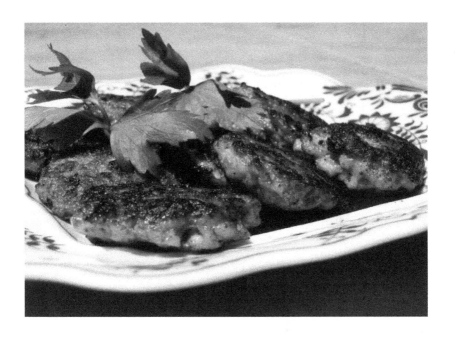

3 Feta Frittata

Preparation Time: 15 minutes

Cooking Time: 15 minutes

Servings: 2

Ingredients:

1 green onion (sliced)

1 clove of garlic (minced)

2 large eggs

½ cup egg substitute

4 tbsps feta cheese (crumbled)

1/3 cup plum tomato (chopped)

4 slices avocado (peeled)

2 tbsp sour cream

Directions:

Heat oil in an iron skillet. Add garlic and onion. Sauté for three minutes.

Combine egg substitute, eggs, and three tablespoons of feta cheese in a bowl. Add the egg mixture to the skillet.

Cook for six minutes.

Sprinkle remaining feta and tomato on top.

Cover and cook for two minutes.

Let the egg rest for five minutes.

Serve with sour cream and avocado.

Nutrition Facts: Calories: 205.3; Protein: 19.3 g; Carbs: 6.7 g; Fat: 12.5 g; Fiber: 3.6 g

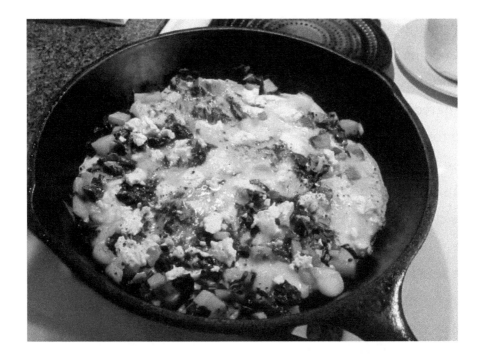

4 Ham Steak with Bacon, Mushrooms, and Gruyere

Preparation Time: 25 minutes

Cooking Time: 10 minutes

Servings: 4

Ingredients:

2 tbsp butter

½ lb mushrooms (sliced)

1 shallot (chopped)

2 cloves garlic (minced)

1/8 tsp black pepper (ground)

1 boneless ham steak (cooked, cut in four equal pieces)

1 cup gruyere cheese (shredded)

4 strips bacon (cooked, crumbled)

1 tbsp parsley (minced)

Directions:

Heat butter in a large iron skillet. Add shallot and mushrooms. Cook the mixture for six minutes. Mix garlic and pepper. Sauté for two minutes. Keep aside.

Cook the ham in the same skillet. Add bacon and cheese. Cook for two minutes.

Serve the ham with the mushroom mixture from the top.

Nutrition: Calories: 356.3; Protein: 35.4 g; Carbs: 5.1 g; Fat: 23.2 g; Fiber: 1.1 g

5 Mushroom-Mascarpone Frittata

Preparation Time: 25 minutes

Cooking Time: 20 minutes

Servings: 6

Ingredients:

8 large eggs

1/3 cup of whipping cream

1/2 cup of Romano cheese (grated)

2 tsp salt

5 tbsp olive oil

¾ lb fresh mushrooms (sliced)

1 onion (sliced)

2 tbsp basil (minced)

2 cloves garlic (minced)

1/8 tsp of pepper

8 oz of mascarpone cheese

Directions:

Whisk together cream, eggs, one-fourth cup of Romano cheese, and salt in a bowl.

Heat two tablespoons of oil in a pan. Add mushrooms and onion. Sauté for two minutes. Add garlic, basil, along with pepper. Stir for one minute. Remove from heat. Add Romano cheese and mascarpone cheese.

Heat one tablespoon of oil in the same pan. Add half mixture of eggs to the pan. Keep cooking for seven minutes. Repeat with the remaining egg mixture.

Place one egg frittata on a plate. Add the mixture of mushrooms. Spread properly.

Add the other layer of the frittata.

Cut in wedges.

Serve immediately.

Nutrition: Calories: 469.3 | Protein: 18.7 g | Carbs: 5.7 g| Fat: 45.4 g | Fiber: 1.6 g

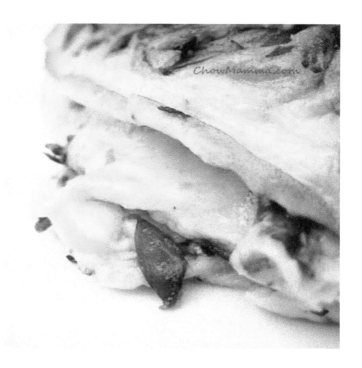

6 Broccoli Quiche Cups

Preparation Time: 5 minutes

Cooking Time: 20 minutes

Servings: 6

Ingredients:

1 cup broccoli (chopped)

1½ cup pepper jack cheese (shredded)

6 large eggs

¾ cup whipping cream

½ cup of bacon bits

1 shallot (minced)

¼ tsp of pepper

¼ tsp of salt

Directions:

Preheat your oven at one-hundred and 70°C.

Divide the cheese and chopped broccoli among twelve greased muffin cups.

Combine the remaining ingredients in a bowl. Divide the prepared mixture among the cups.

Bake the quiche cups for twenty minutes.

Serve immediately.

Nutrition: Calories: 292.3; Protein: 17.6 g; Carbs: 3.6 g; Fat: 25.4 g; Fiber: 0.7 g

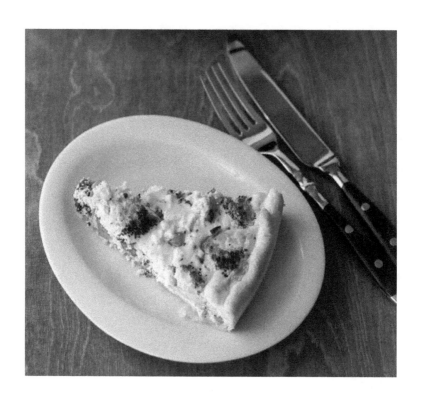

7 Savory Chicken Sausage-Apple

Preparation Time: 10 minutes

Cooking Time: 15 minutes

Servings: 4

Ingredients:

1 tart apple (peeled, diced)

2 tsp poultry seasoning

1 tsp salt

¼ tsp of pepper

1 lb chicken (ground)

Directions:

Take a large bowl. Mix the first four ingredients. Crumble the chicken over the apple mixture. Combine well. Shape the mixture into eight equal patties of three-inch thickness.

Heat oil in an iron skillet.

Cook the apple-chicken patties for six minutes on each side.

Serve hot.

Nutrition: Calories: 93.6; Protein: 9.9 g; Carbs: 3.2 g; Fat: 6.5 g; Fiber: 1.2 g

8 Manchego and Shiitake Scramble

Preparation Time: 10 minutes

Cooking Time: 15 minutes

Servings: 8

Ingredients:

2 tbsp olive oil

½ cup sweet red pepper (diced)

1/2 cup onion (diced)

2 cups shiitake mushrooms (sliced)

1 tsp prepared horseradish

8 large eggs (beaten)

1 cup whipping cream

1 cup of Manchego cheese (shredded)

½ tsp of pepper (ground)

½ tsp of kosher salt

Directions:

Heat one tablespoon of oil in an iron skillet. Add red pepper and onion. Cook for three minutes. Cook the mixture for four minutes after adding the mushrooms along with horseradish. Stir for two minutes.

Whisk the remaining ingredients in a bowl with some olive oil. Pour the mixture into the skillet.

Cook and scramble the eggs for four minutes.

Serve hot.

Nutrition: Calories: 143 Cal; Fat: 11.23 g; Protein: 7.22 g; Carbs: 3.34 g

9 Three-Cheese Quiche

Preparation Time: 10 minutes

Cooking Time: 1 hour

Servings: 6

Ingredients:

7 large eggs

5 egg yolks

1 cup of whipping cream

1 cup of half and half cream

1 cup of mozzarella cheese (shredded)

¾ cup of cheddar cheese (shredded)

½ cup of Swiss cheese (shredded)

2 tbsp of sun-dried tomatoes

1½ tsp of seasoning blend

¼ tsp of basil (dried)

Directions:

Preheat your oven at 150°C.

Combine egg yolks, eggs, whipping cream, mozzarella cheese, half and half cream, half cup of cheddar cheese, tomatoes, Swiss cheese, basil, and seasoning blend in a greased pie dish.

Sprinkle the remaining cheddar cheese on the top.

Bake for 50 minutes.

Let the quiche sit for 10 minutes.

Cut in triangles and serve.

Nutrition: Calories: 448.3; Protein: 21.2 g; Carbs: 5.2 g; Fat: 38.6 g; Fiber: 0.2 g

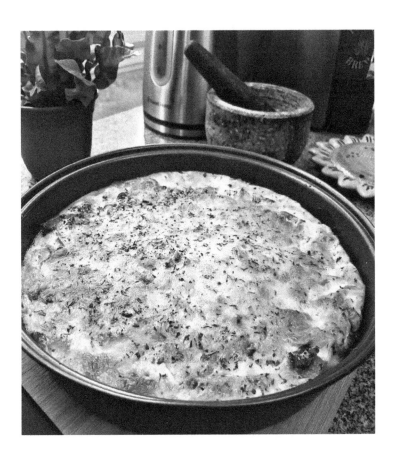

10 Breakfast Turkey Sausage

Preparation Time: 10 minutes

Cooking Time: 12 minutes

Servings: 8

Ingredients:

1 lb lean turkey (ground)

¾ tsp salt

½ tsp rubbed sage

¼ tsp ginger (ground)

1/3 tsp pepper (ground)

Directions:

Crumble the turkey meat in a large bowl. Add sage, salt, ginger, and pepper. Shape the mixture into eight equal patties of two-inch thickness.

Grease an iron skillet with oil.

Add the patties. Cook for six minutes on each side.

Nutrition Facts: Calories: 87.6; Protein: 11.3 g; Carbs: 0.2 g; Fat: 7.5 g; Fiber: 0.1 g

11 No-Bread Breakfast Sandwich

Preparation Time: 7 minutes

Cooking Time: 8 minutes

Servings: 2

Ingredients:

2 tbsp butter

4 large eggs

Pepper and salt

1 oz deli ham (smoked)

2 oz cheddar cheese (cut in slices)

Few drops of Tabasco

Directions:

Heat the butter in an iron skillet. Add the eggs. Fry each side for two minutes. Add pepper and salt.

Take a fried egg. Add ham and cheese. Top with another fried egg.

Repeat for the other fried eggs.

Place the sandwich in the pan for one minute.

Sprinkle some Tabasco on top.

Serve hot.

Nutrition: Calories: 356.3; Protein: 20.3 g; Carbs: 2.1 g; Fat: 31.1 g; Fiber: 0.2 g

12 Baked Eggs

Preparation Time: 5 minutes

Cooking Time: 15 minutes

Servings: 1

Ingredients:

3 oz beef (ground)

2 large eggs

2 oz of cheese (shredded)

Directions:

Preheat your oven at 200°C.

Arrange the ground beef as the base in a baking dish.

Make two holes in the beef base. Crack the eggs in the holes.

Sprinkle cheese on top.

Bake for 15 minutes.

Let the baked eggs rest for 5 minutes.

Nutrition Facts: Calories: 497.6; Protein: 42.1 g; Carbs: 2.1 g; Fat: 34.5 g; Fiber: 0.3 g

13 Cured Salmon with Chives and Scrambled Eggs

Preparation Time: 7 minutes

Cooking Time: 8 minutes

Servings: 2

Ingredients:

2 large eggs

2 tbsp butter

¼ cup whipping cream

1 tbsp chives (chopped)

2 oz cured salmon

Pepper and salt

Directions:

Begin with whisking the eggs in a bowl.

Heat the butter in a pan. Add the eggs. Add the cream. Stir for three minutes.

Simmer for five minutes. Keep stirring to makw the eggs creamy.

Add salt, chopped chives, and pepper.

Serve the eggs with cured salmon.

Nutrition Facts: Calories: 730.2; Protein: 49.6 g; Carbs: 2.1 g; Fat: 61.3 g; Fiber: 0.1 g

14 Eggs Benedict on Avocados

Preparation Time: 10 minutes

Cooking Time: 10 minutes

Servings: 4

Ingredients:

For the hollandaise:

3 egg yolks

1 tbsp of lemon juice

Pepper and salt

8 tbsp of butter (unsalted)

For the eggs:

2 avocados (pitted, skinned)

4 large eggs

5 oz salmon (smoked)

Directions:

Add the butter to a bowl. Microwave for twenty seconds.
Add lemon juice and egg yolks. Use a hand blender for
properly blending the mixture. Keep blending until a white
layer forms. Add pepper and salt. Blend for two minutes.
Boil water in a saucepan. Crack the eggs in a small cup by
cracking one egg at a time. Slide the eggs gently into the water.
Cook for four minutes.
Cut the avocados in half. Add an egg on top of each avocado
slice. Add hollandaise sauce on top.
Add smoked salmon as the side.
Serve immediately.

Nutrition Facts: Calories: 523.6; Protein: 17.6 g; Carbs: 3.1 g; Fat: 49.3 g; Fiber: 7.1 g

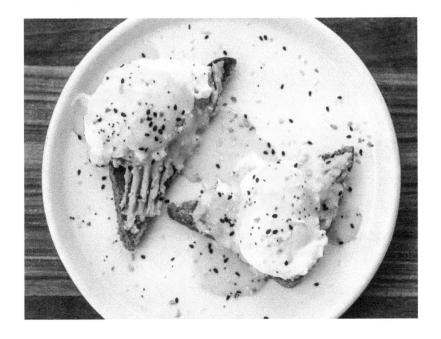

15 Keto Chaffles

Preparation Time: 4 minutes

Cooking Time: 6 minutes

Servings: 4

Ingredients:

1 oz butter (melted)

4 large eggs

8 oz of mozzarella cheese (shredded)

4 tbsp of almond flour

A pinch of salt

Directions:

Preheat a waffle maker.

Mix all the ingredients that have been listed in a mixing bowl. Combine well.

Use butter to grease the waffle maker.

Add one spoonful of the batter to the waffle maker. Close the waffle maker. Cook for six minutes.

Serve immediately with toppings of your choice.

Nutrition: Calories: 332.3; Protein: 23.2 g; Carbs: 1.9 g; Fat: 28.6 g; Fiber: 0.2 g

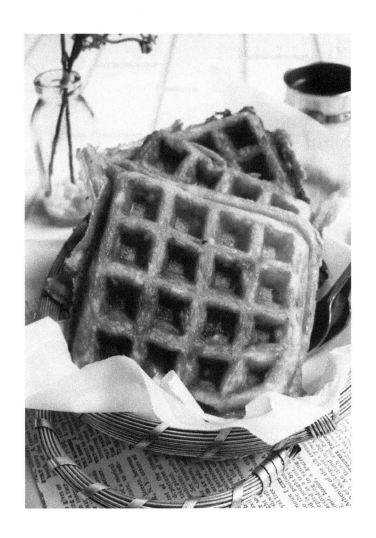

Lunch Recipes

1 Melt-in-Your-Mouth Ribs

Preparation Time: 30 minutes

Cooking Time: 4 hours

Servings: 4

Ingredients:

1½ lb spare ribs

1 tbsp olive oil, at room temperature

2 cloves garlic, chopped

1 Italian pepper, chopped

Salt and black peppercorns to taste

½ tsp ground cumin

2 bay leaves

A bunch of green onions, chopped

¾ cup beef bone broth, preferably homemade

2 tsp erythritol

Directions:

Heat the olive oil in a saucepan over medium-high heat. Sear the ribs for 6-7 minutes on each side.

Whisk the broth, erythritol, garlic, Italian pepper, green onions, salt, pepper, and cumin until well combined.

Place the spare ribs in your crockpot; pour in the pepper/broth mixture. Add in the bay leaves. Cook for about 4 hours on the low setting.

Storage

Divide the pork ribs into four portions. Place each portion of ribs along with the cooking juices in an airtight container; store in your refrigerator for 3-5 days.

To freeze, place the ribs in airtight containers or heavy-duty freezer bags. Freeze for up to 4 to 6 months. Defrost in the refrigerator. Reheat in your oven at 250°F until heated through. Bon appétit!

Nutrition: 412 Calories; 14 g Fat; 4.3 g Carbs; 43.3 g Protein; 0.7 g Fiber

2 Mom's Meatballs in Creamy Sauce

Preparation Time: 5 minutes

Cooking Time: 25 minutes

Servings: 6

Ingredients:

For the Meatballs:

2 eggs

1 tbsp steak seasoning

1 tbsp green garlic, minced

1 tbsp scallions, minced

1 lb ground pork

1/2 lb ground turkey

For the Sauce:

3 tsp ghee

1 cup double cream

1 cup cream of onion soup

Salt and pepper to your liking

½ tsp dried rosemary

Directions:

Preheat your oven to 365°F.

In a mixing bowl, combine all ingredients for the meatballs.
Roll the mixture into 20 to 24 balls and place them on a
parchment-lined baking sheet.

Roast for about 25 minutes or until your meatballs are golden-
brown on the top.

While your meatballs are roasting, melt the ghee in a preheated sauté pan over a moderate flame. Gradually add in the remaining ingredients, whisking constantly, until the sauce has reduced slightly.

Storage

Place the meatballs along with the sauce in airtight containers or Ziploc bags; keep in your refrigerator for up to 3-4 days. Freeze the meatballs in the sauce in airtight containers or heavy-duty freezer bags. Freeze for up to 3-4 months. Reheat on the stove pot or in your oven. Bon appétit!

Nutrition: 378 Calories; 29.9 g Fat; 2.9 g Carbs; 23.4 g Protein; 0.3 g Fiber

3 Mexican-Style Pork Chops

Preparation Time: 15 minutes

Cooking Time: 30 minutes

Servings: 6

Ingredients:

2 Mexican chilies, chopped

1 tsp dried Mexican oregano

½ tsp red pepper flakes, crushed

Salt and ground black pepper, to taste

6 pork chops

½ cup chicken stock

2 garlic cloves, minced

2 tbsp vegetable oil

Directions:

Heat 1 tablespoon of the olive oil in a frying pan over moderate to high heat. Brow the pork chops for 5-6 minutes per side. Then, bring the Mexican chilies and chicken stock to a boil; remove from the heat and let it sit for about 20 minutes. Puree the chilies along with the liquid and the remaining ingredients in your food processor. Add in the remaining oil.

Storage

Divide the pork chops and sauce into six portions; place each portion in a separate airtight container or Ziploc bag; keep in your refrigerator for 3-4 days.

Freeze the pork chops in sauce in airtight containers or heavy-duty freezer bags. Freeze for up to 4 months. Defrost in the refrigerator and reheat in a saucepan. Bon appétit!

Nutrition: 356 Calories; 20.3 g Fat; 0.3 g Carbs; 45.2 g Protein; 0 g Fiber

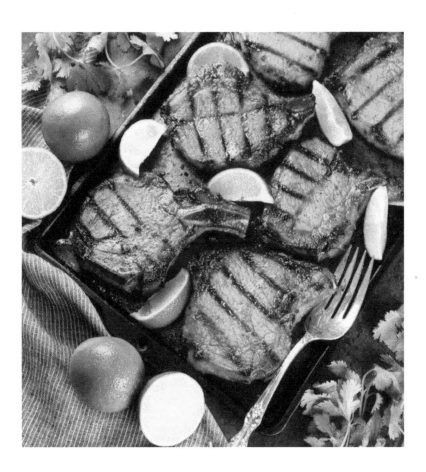

4 Easy Pork Tenderloin Gumbo

Preparation Time: 15 minutes

Cooking Time: 35 minutes

Servings: 6

Ingredients:

1 lb pork tenderloin, cubed

8 oz New Orleans spicy sausage, sliced

1 tbsp Cajun spice mix

1 medium-sized leek, chopped

2 tbsp olive oil

5 cups bone broth

½ cup celery, chopped

1 tsp gumbo file

¼ cup flaxseed meal

¾ lb okra

2 bell peppers, de-veined and thinly sliced

Directions:

In a heavy-bottomed pot, heat the oil until sizzling. Sear the pork tenderloin and New Orleans sausage for about 8 minutes or until browned on all sides; set aside.

In the same pot, cook the leek and peppers until they softened. Add in the gumbo file, Cajun spice, and broth. Bring it to a rolling boil.

Turn the heat to medium-low and add in celery. Let it simmer for 18-20 minutes.

Stir in the flaxseed meal and okra along with the reserved meat. Then, continue to simmer for 5-6 minutes or until heated through.

Storage

Spoon your gumbo into six airtight containers; keep in your refrigerator for up to 3-4 days.

For freezing, place the chilled gumbo in airtight containers or heavy-duty freezer bags. Freeze for up to 5 months. Defrost in the refrigerator and reheat on the stove pot. Enjoy!

Nutrition: 427 Calories; 16.2 g Fat; 3.6 g Carbs; 33.2 g Protein; 4.4 g Fiber

5 Pork and Carrot Mini Muffins

Preparation Time: 15 minutes

Cooking Time: 35 minutes

Servings: 6

Ingredients:

1 egg, whisked

1 oz envelope onion soup mix

Kosher salt and ground black pepper, to taste

2 cloves of garlic, minced

1 cup carrots, shredded

1 cup tomato puree

1 tbsp coconut aminos

1 tbsp stone-ground mustard

1½ tsp dry basil

1 cup Romano cheese, grated

1 lb pork, ground

½ lb turkey, ground

Directions:

In a mixing bowl, combine all ingredients until everything is well incorporated. Press the mixture into a lightly oiled muffin tin.

Bake in the preheated oven at 355°F for 30-33 minutes; let it cool slightly before unmolding and serving.

Storage

Wrap the meatloaf muffins tightly with heavy-duty aluminum foil or plastic wrap. Keep in your refrigerator for up to 3 to 4 days.

For freezing, wrap the meatloaf muffins tightly to prevent freezer burn. They will maintain the best quality for 3-4 months. Defrost in the refrigerator. Bon appétit!

Nutrition: 303 Calories; 17 g Fat; 6.2 g Carbs; 29.6 g Protein; 1.7 g Fiber

6 Bacon Blue Cheese Fat Bombs

Preparation Time: 5 minutes

Cooking Time: 5 minutes

Servings: 4

Ingredients:

1½ tbsp mayonnaise

½ cup bacon, chopped

3 oz blue cheese, crumbled

3 oz cream cheese

2 tbsp chives, chopped

2 tsp tomato puree

Directions:

Mix all ingredients until everything is well combined.

Shape the mixture into 8 equal fat bombs.

Storage

Place the fat bombs in airtight containers or Ziploc bags; keep in your refrigerator for 10 days.

To freeze, arrange the fat bombs on a baking tray in a single layer; freeze for about 2 hours. Transfer the frozen bombs to an airtight container. Freeze for up to 2 months. Serve chilled! Nutrition: 232 Calories; 17.6 g Fat; 2.9 g Carbs; 14.2 g Protein; 0.6 g Fiber

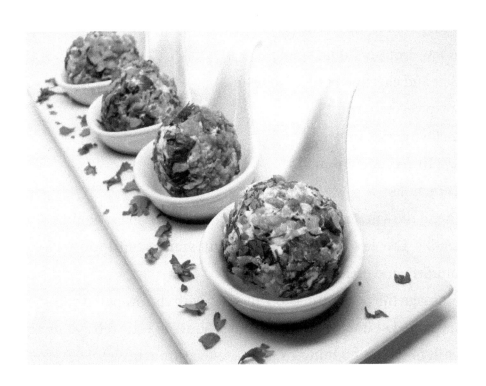

7 Creole-Style Pork Shank

Preparation Time: 2 hours (marinating time)

Cooking Time: 30 minutes

Servings: 6

Ingredients:

1½ lb pork shank, cut into 6 serving portions

1 tbsp Creole seasoning

A few drops of liquid smoke

Salt and cayenne pepper, to taste

3 tsp vegetable oil

2 clove garlic, minced

1½ tbsp coconut aminos

Directions:

Blend the salt, cayenne pepper, vegetable oil, garlic, liquid smoke, Creole seasoning, and coconut aminos until you get a uniform and creamy mixture.

Massage the pork shanks on all sides with the prepared rub mixture. Let it marinate for about 2 hours in your refrigerator. Grill for about 20 minutes until cooked through.

Storage

Put the pork shanks into six airtight containers or Ziploc bags; keep in your refrigerator for 3-4 days.

To freeze, wrap tightly with heavy-duty aluminum foil or freezer wrap. It will maintain the best quality for about 3 months. Defrost in the refrigerator and reheat in your oven. Enjoy!

Nutrition: 335 Calories; 24.3 g Fat; 0.8 g Carbs; 26.4 g
Protein; 0.4 g Fiber

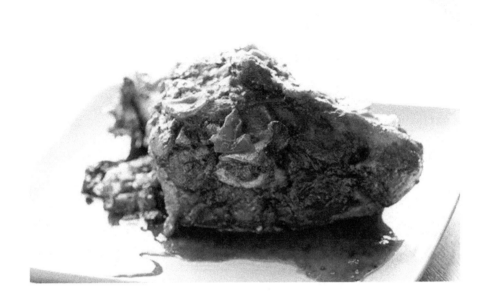

8 German Pork Rouladen

Preparation Time: 2 hours (marinating time)

Cooking Time: 1 hour

Servings: 6

Ingredients:

1½ lb boneless pork loin, butterflied

2 garlic cloves, pressed

1 tbsp ghee, room temperature

1 tbsp Mediterranean herb mix

1 tsp mustard seeds

½ tsp cumin seeds

1 cup roasted vegetable broth

1 large-sized onion, thinly sliced

Salt and black peppercorns, to taste

½ cup Burgundy wine

Directions:

Boil the pork loin for about 5 minutes; pat it dry.

Now, combine the Mediterranean herb mix, mustard seeds, cumin seeds, garlic, and ghee.

Unfold the pork loin and spread the rub all over the cut side.

Roll the pork and secure with kitchen string. Allow it to sit at least 2 hours in your refrigerator.

Place the pork loin in a lightly greased baking pan. Add on wine, broth, onion, salt, and black peppercorns.

Roast in the preheated oven at 390°F for approximately 1 hour.

Storage

Divide the pork and sauce between six airtight containers or Ziploc bags; keep in your refrigerator for up to 3 to 5 days. For freezing, place the pork and sauce in airtight containers or heavy-duty freezer bags. Freeze for up to 4 months. Defrost in the refrigerator and reheat in your oven. Bon appétit!

Nutrition: 220 Calories; 6 g Fat; 2.8 g Carbs; 33.3 g Protein; 0.4 g Fiber

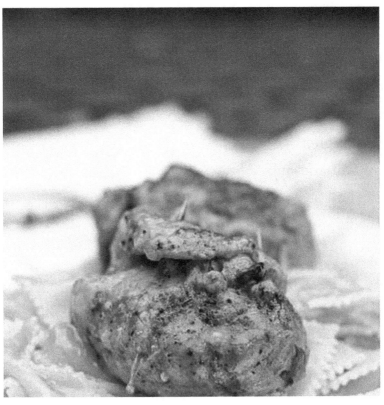

9 Rich Pork and Bacon Meatloaf

Preparation Time: 20 minutes

Cooking Time: 1 hour 10 minutes

Servings: 6

Ingredients:

1¼ lb ground pork

½ lb pork sausage, broken up

6 strips bacon

2 garlic cloves, finely minced

1 tsp celery seeds

Salt and cayenne pepper, to taste

1 bunch coriander, roughly chopped

1 egg, beaten

2 oz half-and-half

1 tsp lard

1 medium-sized leek, chopped

Directions:

Melt the lard in a frying pan over medium-high heat. Cook the leek and garlic until they have softened or about 3 minutes. Add in the ground pork and sausage; cook until it is no longer pink, about 3 minutes. Add in the half-and-half, celery seeds, salt, cayenne pepper, coriander, and egg.

Press the mixture into a loaf pan.

Place the bacon strips on top of your meatloaf and bake at 390°F for about 55 minutes.

Storage

Wrap your meatloaf tightly with heavy-duty aluminum foil or plastic wrap. Store in your refrigerator for up to 3-4 days.

For freezing, wrap your meatloaf tightly to prevent freezer burn. Freeze for up to 3-4 months. Defrost in the refrigerator and reheat in your oven. Bon appétit!

Nutrition: 396 Calories; 24.1 g Fat; 5.1 g Carbs; 38.1 g Protein; 0.5 g Fiber

10 Pork and Vegetable Souvlaki

Preparation Time: 2 hours

Cooking Time: 20 minutes

Servings: 6

Ingredients:

1 tbsp Greek spice mix

2 cloves garlic, crushed

3 tbsp coconut aminos

3 tbsp olive oil

1 tbsp stone-ground mustard

2 tbsp fresh lemon juice

1 lb brown mushrooms

2 bell peppers, cut into thick slices

1 red bell pepper, cut into thick slices

1 zucchini, cubed

1 shallot, cut into wedges

2 lb pork butt, cubed

Bamboo skewers, soaked in cold water for 30 minutes

Directions:

Mix the Greek spice mix, garlic, coconut aminos, olive oil, mustard, and lemon juice in a ceramic dish; add in pork cubes and let it marinate for 2 hours.

Thread the pork cubes and vegetables onto the soaked skewers. Salt to taste.

Grill for about 15 minutes, basting with the reserved marinade.

Storage

Divide the pork and vegetables between six airtight containers or Ziploc bags; keep in your refrigerator for up to 3 to 5 days. For freezing, place the pork and vegetables in airtight containers or heavy-duty freezer bags. Freeze for up to 4 months. Defrost in the refrigerator. Bon appétit!

Nutrition: 267 Calories; 10.6 g Fat; 5.3 g Carbs; 34.9 g Protein; 1.3 g Fiber

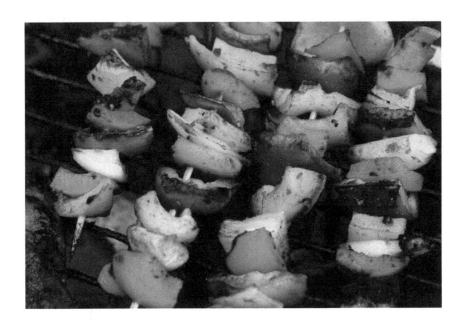

11 Pork Cutlets with Kale

Preparation Time: 2 hours (marinating time)

Cooking Time: 25 minutes

Servings: 6

Ingredients:

Sea salt and ground black pepper, to taste

2 tsp olive oil

¼ cup port wine

2 garlic cloves, smashed

2 tbsp oyster sauce

2 tbsp fresh lime juice

1 medium leek, sliced

2 bell peppers, chopped

2 cups kale

1½ lb pork cutlets

Directions:

Sprinkle the pork with salt and black pepper. Then, make the marinade by whisking one teaspoon of olive oil, wine, garlic, oyster sauce, and lime juice.

Let the pork marinate for about 2 hours in your refrigerator

Heat the remaining tsp of olive oil in a frying pan. Fry the leek and bell peppers for 4 to 5 minutes, stirring continuously until they have softened slightly; set aside.

In the same pan, sear the pork along with the marinade until browned on all sides.

Stir the reserved vegetables into the frying pan along with the kale. Continue to cook for 5 to 6 minutes more.

Storage

Place the pork chops and vegetables in airtight containers or Ziploc bags; keep in your refrigerator for 3 to 4 days.

Freeze the pork chops and vegetables in airtight containers or heavy-duty freezer bags. Freeze for up to 4 months. Defrost in the refrigerator. Bon appétit!

Nutrition: 234 Calories; 11 g Fat; 2 g Carbs; 29.8 g Protein; 0.9 g Fiber

12 Italian Keto Plate

Take your mind off of work for a bit and take your imagination to Italy with this amazing dish.

Preparation Time: 5 minutes

Cooking Time: 5 minutes

Servings: 1

Ingredients:

7 oz mozzarella cheese

7 oz fatty Italian deli meat

2 sliced tomatoes

⅓ cup olive oil

10 green or black olives

Salt and pepper to taste

Directions:

Put all of the ingredients on a plate or in your lunch tin. Serve with olive oil, and spice with salt & pepper to taste.

Nutrition: Carbohydrates: 24.7 g; Fat: 133 g; Protein: 108 g

13 Steak Tartare

You can have a themed lunch, almost every day with our cookbook. This wholesome Steak Tartare recipe will take you to France.

Preparation Time: 5 minutes

Cooking Time: 15 minutes

Servings: 2

Ingredients:

10 oz ground fatty beef cuts

2 tbsp capers

2 tbsp mild mustard

2 tbsp parmesan cheese

1 tbsp horseradish

2 separated eggs

1 cup baby lettuce

2 oz bottled chopped beetroot

Salt and pepper to taste

Directions:

Grate the horseradish and parmesan cheese. Wash and dry the lettuce, then arrange it on the plates.

Divide the ground, fatty beef into two equal parts. Form a patty and arrange it in the middle of the plate. Push an indentation in the middle of the patty with the back of a spoon. Arrange the rest of the vegetables around the patty and on top of the lettuce.

Gently spoon the egg yolks on top of the patty. Season well with salt and pepper.

Nutrition: Carbohydrates: 7.2 g; Fat: 15.7 g; Protein: 50.1 g

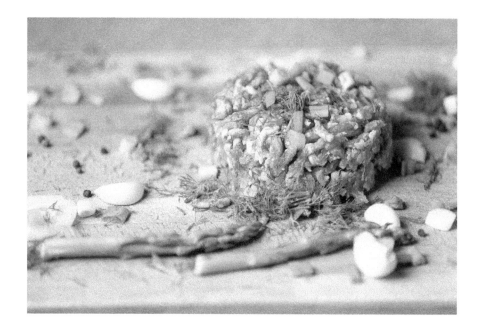

14 Keto Deviled Eggs

Doesn't this recipe take you back to lazy weekends in the park, reading a book, and having a picnic?

Cooking Time: 10 minutes

Preparation Time: 5 minutes

Cooking Time: 10 minutes

Servings: 4

Ingredients:

4 hard-boiled eggs, shelled and halved

1 tsp Tabasco sauce

¼ cup full-fat mayo

8 cooked and peeled shrimp

Salt and pepper to taste

Directions:

Scoop out the yolk from the eggs and put the egg whites on a plate, with the hollowed sides pointing upwards.

In a bowl, mash the yolks. Then add Tabasco sauce, spices, and mayonnaise.

Spoon the mixture back into the hollowed egg whites and place a shrimp on top of the mixture.

Nutrition: Carbohydrates: 4.5 g; Fat: 10 g; Protein: 15.7 g

15 Oven-baked Brie Cheese

For the love of cheese! Who can disa-brie?

Cooking Time: 5 minutes

Preparation Time: 10 minutes

Cooking Time: 5 minutes

Servings: 1

Salmon Ingredients:

9 oz camembert or brie cheese wedge

1 peeled and crushed garlic clove

1 tbsp dried rosemary

2 oz pecan & walnuts mixed

1 tbsp extra virgin olive oil

Salt and pepper to taste

Directions:

Preheat the oven to 400°F.

Remove the wrapping from the cheese wedge. Place the whole cheese wedge on a baking sheet lined with foil or parchment paper.

Combine the remainder of the additives in a small mixing bowl, and mix well.

Place the mixture on top of the cheese wedge and place it in the oven.

Bake the cheese for a period of 10 minutes, remove out of the oven and serve immediately.

Nutrition: Carbohydrates: 12.4 g; Fat: 116.9 g; Protein: 56.9 g

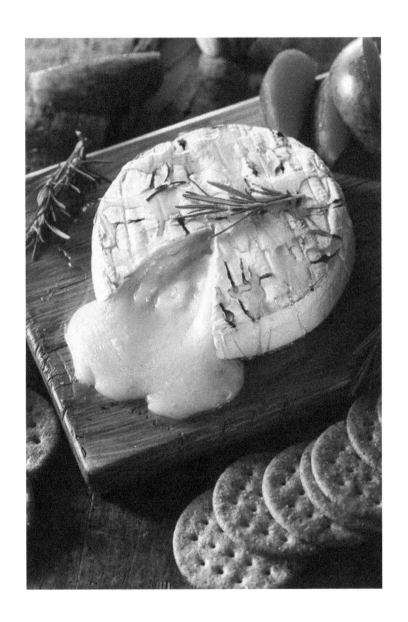

Dinner Recipes

1   Keto Taco Cups

All the flavors of Mexico, in the palm of your hand, ready for you to enjoy.

Preparation Time: 10 minutes

Cooking Time: 20 minutes

Servings: 12

Ingredients:

2 cups grated parmesan cheese

1 tbsp olive oil

1 tbsp of garlic paste

1 small red onion, diced

1 lb ground (minced) fatty pork meat

1 tbsp smoked paprika spice

1 tbsp chili powder

1 tbsp cumin

Salt, pepper, and other aromatics, to taste

Tub of sour cream for serving

Chopped avocado, tomatoes, and coriander for serving

Directions:

Cut parchment paper (wax paper) into 12 squares of equal size. This will aid in transferring the cheese to the muffin tin.

Prepare a 12-inch regular muffin pan, and lightly coat with cooking spray or brush the edges of each individual tin with 2 tbsp of melted, unsalted butter.

Preheat the oven to 375°F, and line a baking sheet with the 12 prepared squares of parchment paper.

Place two tablespoons of parmesan cheese onto each individual piece of parchment paper. Ensure that the squares are about 2-3 inches apart.

Bake the cheese in the oven until the edges turn brown in color. Take out of the oven, and allow to cool for a few minutes.

Place a piece of baked cheese into each muffin tin, and use your hands to gently mold the cheese around the edges and the bottom of each tin cup.

In a sizable skillet, fire up the olive oil over medium heat. Add the onion and brown until soft. Next, add the garlic paste and minced pork meat. Cook the pork until it's not pink anymore. Add the desired seasoning to the pan of meat. Place the baked cheese cups on a platter, and spoon the cooked meat into each cup.

Top with the avocado, coriander, tomato, and sour cream.

Nutrition: Carbohydrates: 1.6 g; Fat: 4.6 g; Protein: 12.7 g

2 Loaded Cauliflower Salad

All the crunch from the cauliflower florets and stuff with mouthfuls of cheese and fragrant, crunchy bacon bits.

Preparation Time: 10 minutes

Cooking Time: 30 minutes

Servings: 6

Ingredients:

1 large head of cauliflower, washed and cut into florets

¼ cup water

½ cup crispy bacon bits

½ sour cream

¼ full fat mayo

1 tbsp lemon juice

1½ grated cheddar cheese

¼ cup finely diced chives

Salt, pepper, and other aromatics, to taste

Directions:

Bring the water to a boil on the stove in a large pot or saucepan. Add the cauliflower florets to the pot, steam for 4 minutes. Drain the florets on a paper towel.

In a small frying pan, fry the bacon until crispy.

Combine the mayo, sour cream, and lemon juice in a large mixing bowl, and whisk well together. Add the cauliflower florets, and fold gently together.

Season well with the desired spices. Fold in the cheddar, chives, and bacon. Serve.

Nutrition: Carbohydrates: 13 g; Fat: 35 g; Protein: 19 g

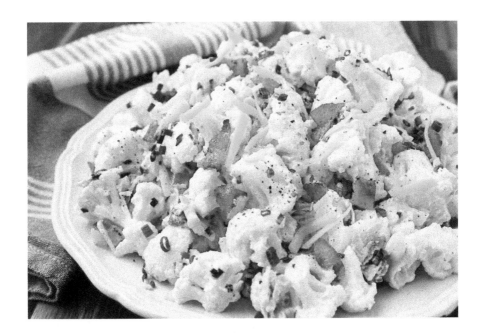

3 Caprese Zoodles

Pasta can be healthy too when replacing the pasta with actual vegetable strips.

Preparation Time: 10 minutes

Cooking Time: 15 minutes

Servings: 4

Ingredients:

4 large, washed baby marrows (zucchini)

2 tbsp olive oil

2 cups cocktail tomatoes, cut lengthwise

1 cup mozzarella cheese balls

¼ cup basil leaves

2 tbsp red wine vinegar

Salt, pepper, and other aromatics, to taste

Directions:

Make zoodles from the baby marrow by turning and pushing it through a spiralizer tool.

In a large bowl, coat the fresh zoodles in olive oil, season well, and allow to marinate for 15 minutes. Add tomatoes, cheese, and basil, swirl gently until all of the additives are well-combined.

Dish the required amount on each serving plate. Drizzle with red wine vinegar. Serve.

Nutrition: Carbohydrates: 14.4 g; Fat: 9.5 g; Protein: 6 g

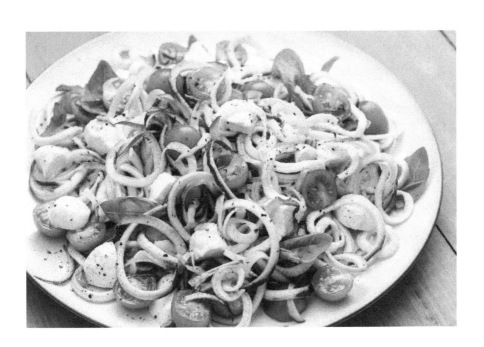

4 Keto Broccoli and Cheddar Soup

Some healthy vegetables, submerged in a luscious bath of cheddar cheese. Comfort at its best.

Preparation Time: 15 minutes

Cooking Time: 25 minutes

Servings: 6

Ingredients:

4 tbsp unsalted butter

1 large carrot, peeled and sliced into thin sticks

2 garlic cloves, peeled and crushed

¾ tbsp sweet, smoked paprika

¾ tbsp mustard powder

¾ tbsp onion powder

4 cups chicken stock or homemade chicken broth

6 cups small broccoli florets

6 oz plain cream cheese

4 cups shredded cheddar cheese

Salt, pepper, and other spices, to taste

Directions:

In a medium-sized skillet, melt the unsalted butter. Then add the carrot and garlic, and cook until the garlic is fragrant. Normally, this takes about 3 minutes.

Next, combine the paprika, mustard, cayenne, and onion powder, and stir well. Add the chicken stock or broth to the mix, and season well.

Add the broccoli florets to the mix and cook for 5 minutes, until tender. Combine the cheddar and cream cheese, and stir continuously until the cheese has melted.

Season if needed, and serve warm.

Nutrition: Carbohydrates: 10.1 g; Fat: 43.5 g; Protein: 24.9 g

5 Egg Roll Bowls

This eating plan is so good to you, that you are even permitted to have your favorite egg rolls. Unleash the flavor!

Preparation Time: 10 minutes

Cooking Time: 25 minutes

Servings: 4

Ingredients:

1 tbsp avocado oil

1 garlic clove, peeled and crushed

1 tbsp ginger

1 lb. ground pork

1 tbsp sesame oil

½ red onion, finely diced

1 cup grated carrot

¼ head of green cabbage, thinly shredded

½ cup low-sodium soy sauce

1 tbsp sriracha paste

1 scallion, finely chopped

1 tbsp mixed seeds (sunflower, poppy, sesame)

Salt, pepper, and other spices, as desired.

Directions:

In a sizable skillet, heat the avocado oil, over medium heat. Add the garlic and ginger to the skillet and cook for 3 minutes, until fragrant. Add the ground pork, cook until the meat no longer has any pink hues.

Move the pork to the one side of the pan. Add the sesame oil, onion, carrot, and cabbage to the same pan. Stir and combine this with the meat. Combine the sriracha paste and soy sauce. Cook for 6-7 minutes, until the cabbage is tender. Transfer to dishes for serving and season to taste. Top with mixed seeds, and scallion.

Nutrition:

Carbohydrates: 11 g; Fat: 32 g; Protein: 22 g

6 Quesadillas - Keto Style

This eating plan is so good to you, that you are even permitted to have your favorite egg rolls. Unleash the flavor!

Preparation Time: 10 minutes

Cooking Time: 25 minutes

Servings: 4

Ingredients:

1 tbsp olive oil

1 bell pepper, diced

⅓ red onion, finely diced

½ tsp chili powder

3 cups parmesan cheese, grated

3 cups smoked chicken, shredded

1 avocado, peeled and thinly diced

1 scallion, finely chopped

3 cups sharp cheddar, grated

Salt, pepper, and other spices, to taste

Tub of sour cream for serving

Directions:

Line two baking sheets with parchment paper (wax paper) and preheat the oven to 400°F.

Heat the olive oil in a medium-sized frying pan. Combine the pepper, red onion, and season well. Cook for 5 minutes until soft, remove from heat, and add to a plate.

In a mixing bowl, combine the cheddar cheese and parmesan cheeses. Scoop 1½ cups of the cheese mixture onto the middle of each lined baking sheet. With a spoon, spread it out into a layer and shape to simulate a flour tortilla.

Transfer to the oven and bake the cheese until the edges turn crispy, and the cheese is melted. Remove from the oven. Add the pepper and onion mixture, chicken, and slices of avocado on one side of each of the tortillas.

Allow to cool for a few minutes, and fold over the side that does not have the filling, into a folded omelet. Return to the oven for 4 minutes. Repeat the process with the leftover cheese.

Cut the quesadilla into quarters, serve with sour cream and scallion.

Nutrition: Carbohydrates: 12.8 g; Fat: 46.7 g; Protein: 99.9 g

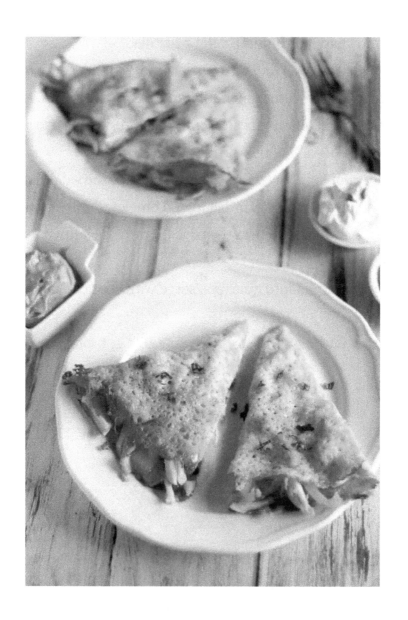

7 Cheeseburger Tomatoes

No one really eats both the buns, right? Now you eat your cheeseburger completely guilt-free.

Preparation Time: 5 minutes

Cooking Time: 20 minutes

Servings: 4

Ingredients:

1 tbsp olive oil

1 medium-sized red onion, diced

2 garlic cloves, peeled and crushed

1 lb ground beef (not lean)

1 tbsp ketchup. Check for a brand that does not have added sugar

1 tbsp keto-friendly mustard

4 medium-sized tomatoes

⅔ cup sharp cheddar, grated

¼ cup spinach, shredded

½ tsp chili powder

4 slices of pickle

Salt, pepper, and other spices, as desired.

Directions:

Fire up the olive oil in a medium-sized skillet over medium heat. Put in the onion, and fry until softened. Join the garlic, and cook for 3 minutes. Add the beef, and cook until the meat is no longer pink. Break the big chunks of beef by breaking it up with a spoon.

Drain the remaining grease in the pan. Season with desired spices. Add ketchup and mustard and stir well.

Wash and dry the tomatoes, and bring them to stand on their stem sides. Cut the tomatoes into 6 equal wedges, but don't cut it all the way through. Gently open the wedges and spoon the beef mixture equally into the 4 tomatoes. Add a slice of pickle on top.

Nutrition: Carbohydrates: 15.4 g; Fat: 20 g; Protein: 37.1 g

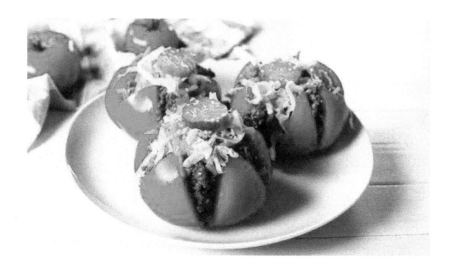

8 Three Cheese Chicken and Cauliflower

Another great alternative to pasta that tastes even better than the original dish.

Preparation Time: 40 minutes

Cooking Time: 1 hour

Servings: 8

Filling Ingredients:

1 tbsp olive oil

1 leek, thinly diced

2 cups ground chicken

1 pt. button mushrooms, washed and sliced

1 packet baby spinach, washed and shredded

1 cup cream cheese

1 tsp tarragon

½ canned tomato paste

1 cup mozzarella cheese, grated

Salt, pepper, and other spices, to taste

Lasagna Sheet Ingredients:

1 large cauliflower head

½ cup parmesan cheese

2 whole eggs

Non-stick spray

Directions:

Heat up the oven to 356°F prior to starting out.

Chop up half of the cauliflower head, and add to a blender or food processor. Chop finely. This can also be done manually by hand, using a sharp knife and cutting board. Move the chopped cauliflower and place it aside in a mixing bowl. Repeat the process with the other half.

Add 2 cups of water. Cover the bowl with cling wrap or a lid, and microwave on a high setting until it's tender, stirring occasionally throughout the cooking process. Once done, drain the excess liquid through a sieve. Return to the bowl and add the parmesan cheese, egg, and season well. Combine the mixture.

Using two baking trays, line them with parchment paper. Divide the mixture equally between the two baking sheets. Use your fingers to press the mixture into the baking sheets in rectangles along the edges. Put in the oven and cook until the mixture has dried out. Take out of the oven and allow to cool. Cut into a width of 10 cm to make lasagna sheets.

Heat the olive oil in a large skillet over high heat. Add the leek, and reduce the heat to low. Cook until soft. Add the chicken, and break the lumps of meat into smaller pieces with a wooden spoon. Cook for at least 5 minutes. Add the mushrooms, and cook for 5 minutes.

Next, add the spinach, and cook until wilted. Add the cream cheese and cook until melted. Stir in the tarragon, and season according to taste.

Coat an oven-proof baking dish with the cooking spray (24-cm top measurement and 19-cm base measurement). Brush the base and the edges of the baking dish with the tomato paste. Place 2 sheets over the tomato paste.

Scoop ½ of the chicken mixture on top and sprinkle with ⅓ cup of mozzarella cheese. Add another layer of cauliflower and repeat the process. End with the remaining tomato paste and mozzarella on top. Bake for 30 minutes in the oven. Take out and allow to rest outside the oven for 7 minutes until firm.

Nutrition: Carbohydrates: 16.1 g; Fat: 19.5 g; Protein: 23. 5 g

9 Garlic Butter Salmon with Lemon Asparagus Skillet

One of the great advantages of this dish is that it is packed with flavor, and can be cooked in one pan. It's one of the quickest dishes to prepare in our cookbook.

Preparation Time: 5 minutes

Cooking Time: 25 minutes

Servings: 2

Filling Ingredients:

1 medium salmon, divided into 4 equal portions

2 bundles of green asparagus, washed and trimmed

1 tbsp extra virgin olive oil

2 tbsp garlic flakes

½ cup dry white wine

110 g of unsalted butter

1 tbsp sriracha sauce

3 oz lemon juice

1 tbsp coriander

1 tbsp parsley

4 lemon cheeks for garnish and drizzle afterward

Salt, pepper, and other spices, to taste

Directions:

Pat the salmon chunks dry on both sides with a kitchen towel, and place them on a cutting board. Season well with desired spices, and rub the spices across the surface of the salmon. Marinate in the salt rub.

In a medium pan, add the asparagus, and add water, until the vegetables are covered, and cook for 2 minutes. Transfer to an ice-water bath immediately after the 3 minutes have elapsed. Heat the olive oil in a non-stick cast-iron skillet over medium heat. Sear the salmon on both sides. Gently flip it over with a spatula each time, so as not to disturb the flaky texture of the fish. Once the salmon is golden brown on both sides, remove from the skillet and transfer to a plate.

In the skillet that the fish was cooked, add the minced garlic and cook for 3 minutes until fragrant. Add the white wine, and reduce the heat to cook the alcohol away. Add the butter, lemon juice, sriracha paste, and parsley. Stir to combine.

Add the asparagus to the pan, and cook for 2 minutes. Add the salmon back into the pan, and reheat. Gently turning the chunks over.

Sprinkle with parsley and add the cheeks of lemon. Serve immediately.

Nutrition: Carbohydrates: 13.51 g; Fat: 38.57 g; Protein: 42.09 g

10 Hearty Shrimp Curry

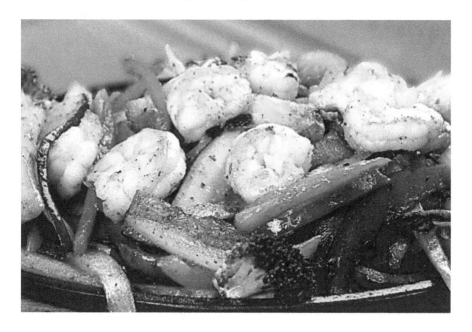

Preparation Time: 5 minutes

Cooking Time: 10 minutes

Servings: 2

Ingredients:

2 tbsp Green Curry paste

1 cup vegetable stock

1 cup coconut milk

6 oz pre-cooked shrimp

5 oz Broccoli florets

3 tbsp chopped cilantro

2 tbsp coconut oil

1 tbsp soy sauce

Juice of half of a lime

1 medium-sized spring onion, chopped

1 tsp crushed roasted garlic

1 tsp minced garlic

1 tsp fish sauce

½ tsp turmeric

¼ tsp Xanthan gum

½ cup sour cream

Directions:

Place a pan over medium heat and add two tablespoons of coconut oil.

Add minced ginger, chopped up onion and cook for a minute.

Add turmeric and curry paste.

Add the soy sauce and fish sauce, and mix.

Add a cup of vegetable stock and a cup of coconut milk.

Stir well and add green curry paste. Simmer.

Add ¼ tsp of Xanthan gum and mix well.

After a while, you will notice that the curry will begin to thicken, that will be the moment when you are going to be needing to add the florets and stir them finely.

Add the fresh chopped cilantro.

Once you have a nice consistency, add the weighed, pre-cooked shrimp and lime juice.

Allow the mix to simmer for a few minutes and season with pepper and salt.

Serve with sour cream.

Enjoy!

Nutrition: Protein: 27 g; Carbs: 8.9 g; Fats: 31 g; Calories: 454

11 Ancient Salmon Glaze and Teriyaki

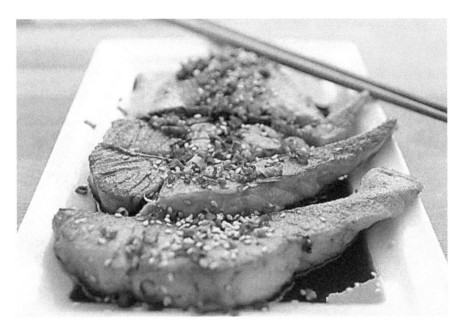

Preparation Time: 10 minutes

Cooking Time: 10 minutes

Servings: 2

Ingredients:

10 oz of salmon fillet

2 tbsp soy sauce

2 tsp sesame oil

1 tbsp rice vinegar

1 tsp minced ginger

2 tsp minced garlic

1 tbsp red boat fish sauce

1 tbsp sugar-free ketchup

2 tbsp dry white wine

Directions:

Toss in all of the ingredients in a small-sized bowl. Just make sure not to toss the sesame oil, white wine, and ketchup.

Marinate for about 10-15 minutes.

Bring down the pan to a nice heat and toss in the sesame oil.

Once the smoke is seen, toss the fish with the skin side down. Let it cook until crispy.

Flip it and cook the other side. Each side should take about 3-4 minutes.

Pour in the marinade into the fish and let it boil.

Slowly remove the fish from the pan and pour in the ketchup alongside the white wine to the liquid in the pan.

Simmer for 5 minutes and serve as a side.

Nutrition: Protein: 33 g; Carbs: 2.5 g; Fats: 23.5 g; Calories: 370

12 Extremely Low Carb Chicken Satay

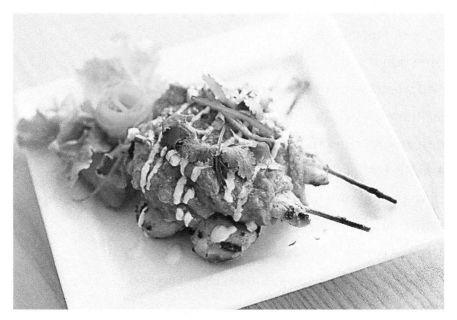

Preparation Time: 5 minutes

Cooking Time: 5 minutes

Servings: 1

Ingredients:

1 lb ground chicken

4 tbsp soy sauce

2 onion springs

1/3 of a yellow pepper

1 tbsp erythritol

1 tbsp rice vinegar

2 tsp sesame oil

2 tsp chili paste

1 tsp minced garlic

1/3 tsp cayenne pepper

¼ tsp paprika

Juice of half a lime

Directions:

Add 2 teaspoons of sesame oil to a pan and heat it over medium-high heat.

Add ground chicken to your pan and allow it to brown.

Add the rest of the ingredients and mix well.

Once the mixture has reached your desired texture, add the spring onions and sliced yellow pepper.

Mix and serve!

Nutrition: Protein: 105 g; Carbs: 18 g; Fats: 69 g; Calories: 1180

13 Spicy Hot Chicken and Pepper Soup

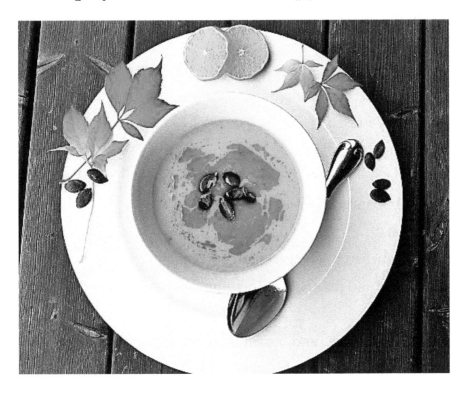

Preparation Time: 5 minutes

Cooking Time: 10 minutes

Servings: 5

Ingredients:

1 tsp coriander seeds

2 tbsp olive oil

2 sliced chili pepper

2 cups chicken broth

2 cups water

1 tsp turmeric

½ tsp ground cumin

4 tbsp tomato paste

16 oz chicken thigh

2 tbsp butter

1 medium-sized avocado

2 oz Queso Fresco

4 tbsp chopped cilantro

Juice of a half lime

Salt and pepper as required

Directions:

Cut the chicken thigh into small portions.

Take a pan and place it over medium heat. Add oil and allow it to heat up.

Add chicken pieces and brown them on both sides. Transfer to a platter and keep it on the side.

Add olive oil to the pan and add coriander seeds. Toast until fragrant.

Pour water and broth, and simmer over low heat.

Season with pepper, turmeric, salt, and ground cumin.

Bring the mix to a simmer. Add tomato paste, butter, and stir well.

Simmer for 10 minutes and add the lime juice.

Add the cooked chicken thigh and mix well.

Garnish with avocado, cilantro, and Queso Fresco.

Enjoy!

Nutrition: Protein: 28 g; Carbs: 10.8 g; Fats: 27 g; Calories: 395

14 Butter Fried Kale and Pork With Cranberries

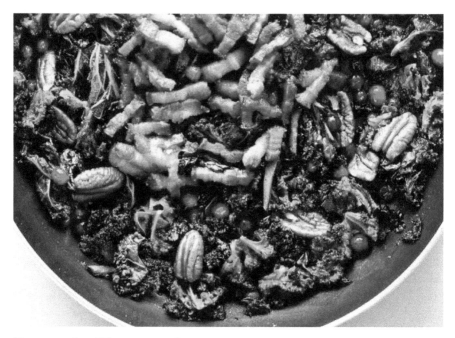

Preparation Time: 10 minutes

Cooking Time: 10 minutes

Servings: 4

Ingredients:

3 oz butter

1 lb kale

¾ lb smoked pork belly

2 oz pecans

½ cup frozen cranberries

Directions:

Rinse, trim and chop your kale into large-sized chunks. Keep it on the side.

Cut the pork belly into strips and fry them in butter over medium-high heat.

Once they are golden brown and crispy, add kale to the pan and fry for a few minutes.

Remove the heat and add cranberries and nuts to the pan. Stir well and serve!

Nutrition: Protein: 21 g; Carbs: 10 g; Fats: 12 g; Calories: 223

15 Amazing Keto Zucchini Hash

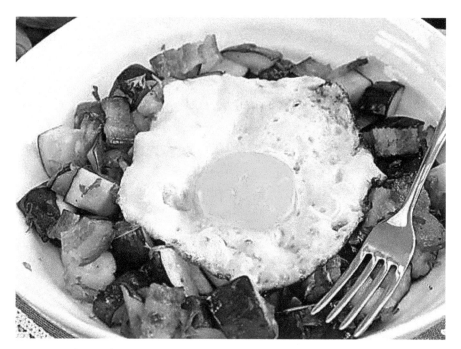

Preparation Time: 10 minutes

Cooking Time: 10-15 minutes

Servings: 4

Ingredients:

1 medium-sized zucchini

2 slices of bacon

½ of a small white onion

1 tbsp coconut oil

1 tbsp freshly chopped parsley

¼ tsp salt

1 large egg

Directions:

Peel and finely chop the onion. Slice the bacon.

Sweat the onions over medium heat and add the bacon. Make sure to stir from time to time to ensure that they are lightly browned.

Dice the zucchini into medium pieces.

Add zucchini to your pan and cook for 10-15 minutes. Remove the heat and add chopped parsley.

Top with a fried egg and enjoy!

Nutrition: Protein: 17 g; Carbs: 6 g; Fats: 35 g; Calories: 423

Poultry Recipes

1 Espetada

Espetada is a traditional dish in Portuguese cuisine that originated in Portugal. It is the technique of making food on skewers, and they are cooked over hot coals or wood chips. However, you can also bake the Espetadas in the oven. They turn out just as delicious.

Preparation Time: 10 minutes + 60 minutes (minimum) marinating time

Cooking Time: 30 minutes

Servings: 4

Ingredients:

8 chicken pieces (drumstick and thighs)

1 cup full cream yogurt

1 tsp Dijon mustard

4 tbsp fresh ginger (grated)

4 tbsp crushed garlic

1 tsp chili flakes (optional)

1 tsp garam masala

½ tsp salt

Ingredients:

You can either make the Espetadas in the oven or barbeque them. If baking them in the oven, preheat the oven to 350°F (180°C).

In a medium-size bowl mix the yogurt, Dijon mustard, ginger, garlic, chili flakes, garam masala, and Himalayan salt.

Place the chicken into the mixture and make sure it covers all of the chicken.

Cover the bowl with cling wrap and place in the refrigerator for at least 1 hour. For best results, place overnight.

If you are using wooden skewers, then soak them in hot water for at least an hour.

Thread the marinated chicken onto the skewers (A thigh and a drumstick on one skewer).

Place the Espetadas into an ovenproof pan and bake for 30 minutes or until done. If barbequing, place the chicken skewers onto the hot grill. Use tongs to turn the skewers occasionally until slightly charred and cooked through, about 20-30 minutes.

Quick Tip: If the juices run clear, the chicken is fully cooked. If the fluid has a slight pink tinge to it, it needs more cooking time.

Nutrition: Fat: 17.3 g; Protein: 31.4 g; Carbs: 7.6 g; Fiber: 0.8 g; Calories: 316

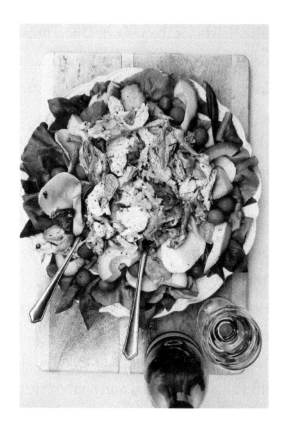

2 Chicken Caprese Salad with Avocado

Preparation Time: 15 minutes

Cooking Time: 20 minutes

Servings: 2

Ingredients:

Olive Oil and Balsamic Vinegar Marinade and Salad Dressing

⅓ cup balsamic vinegar

2 cloves crushed garlic

⅛ tsp black pepper (add more to taste)

½ tsp salt (add more to taste)

1 tbsp Dijon mustard

⅔ cup olive oil

Caprese Salad

2 chicken fillets with skin

1 tbsp butter

2 cups shredded lettuce leaves

½ avocado, sliced

½ cup cherry or Roma tomatoes

½ cup mozzarella (sliced)

1/3 cup basil leaves

Salt and pepper, to taste

Directions:

Start with the marinade/salad dressing first.

Take a medium-sized bowl and mix the balsamic vinegar, garlic, black pepper, salt, Dijon mustard, and olive oil. Taste and add more salt and pepper if necessary.

Take about half of the marinade and put it into a bowl with the chicken. Make sure that all the chicken pieces are covered in the marinade. Marinate for at least 30 minutes.

While the chicken marinates, get started with the salad.

Take a flat salad bowl and arrange the lettuce, avocados, tomatoes, mozzarella, and basil to your liking.

Melt the butter in a medium-sized pan and fry the marinated chicken fillets for about a total of 7 minutes on each side, turning every few minutes until done. Let the chicken rest for about 3 minutes and slice it up (if you prefer your chicken to be cold in the salad, let it cool down completely, then cut it into slices).

Place the chicken on top of the salad and drizzle on the salad dressing.

Quick Tip:

If you want to know whether an avocado is ripe, simply peel back the small stem or cap at the top of the avocado. If it comes away easily and you find green underneath, you've got the perfect avocado that's ripe and ready to eat.

Nutrition: Fat: 70 g; Protein: 68 g; Carbs: 15.6 g; Fiber: 5.1 g; Calories: 967

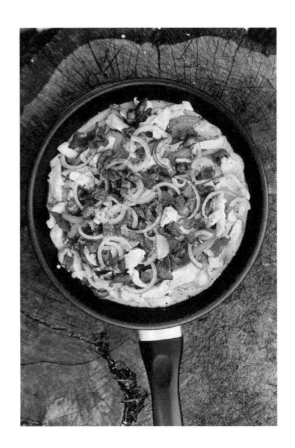

3 Creamy Chicken with Salami and Olives

Preparation Time: 5 minutes

Cooking Time: 30 minutes

Servings: 2

Ingredients:

2 chicken breasts cut into strips. Remove the skin and set aside.

½ onion sliced

½ red bell pepper sliced

1 tsp crushed garlic

10 salami slices cut in quarters (sugar-free)

3 tbsp butter

1 cup chicken stock

½ cup green olives

1 cup cream

Salt and pepper to taste

Method:

In a large pan, melt the butter over medium heat.

Add the onion, bell pepper, garlic, salami, and chicken skin.

Fry until soft and slightly brown.

Add the stock and olives, and reduce by half.

Add the cream and reduce by a third.

Add the chicken pieces and cook until the chicken is cooked.

Season with salt and pepper to taste.

Quick Tip: Letting the salami get to room temperature makes it easier to cut and brings out the best salami flavor. Always check your ingredients to ensure there are no hidden carbs.

Nutrition: Fat: 102.7 g; Protein: 49.8 g; Carbs: 8 g; Fiber: 4.1 g; Calories: 1167

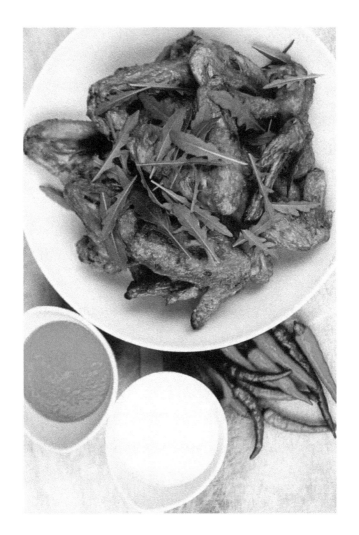

4 Buffalo Wings, Hot Sauce & Blue Cheese Dip

Preparation Time: 15 minutes

Cooking Time: 70 minutes

Servings: 4

Ingredients:

2 lb/1kg chicken wings

2½ tsp baking powder

½ tsp salt

Hot Sauce

Blue Cheese Dip

Directions:

Preheat the oven to 250°F (120°C). Put one oven shelf in the lower quarter of the oven and one in the top quarter.

Pat the chicken dry with paper towels. Place in a medium-size bowl and sprinkle the baking powder and salt over it. Toss well so that the chicken is evenly coated.

Line a tray with foil and place a baking rack on top of it. Place the chicken on the baking rack and place it in the lower quarter of the oven. Bake for 30 minutes.

When done, remove the chicken from the lower quarter and turn the oven up to 425°F/220°C. Put the chicken back in the oven (the top quarter) and bake for another 40 to 50 minutes. The chicken is done when the skin is nice and crispy. Drizzle over some hot sauce and serve with the blue cheese dip.

Quick Tip: The trick to getting your chicken wings ultra-crispy is using baking powder. How exactly does adding baking powder make the wings crispy? When adding the baking powder, the pH level on the skin rises, and this causes the peptide bonds to break down. Now your chicken will be ultra-crispy and golden brown.

Nutrition (Baked Wings): Fat: 48 g; Protein: 67 g; Carbs: 0.7 g; Fiber: 0 g; Calories: 722

Nutrition (Baked Wings with Red Hot Sauce): Fat: 60 g; Protein: 68 g; Carbs: 3.3 g; Fiber: 0.4 g; Calories: 843

Nutrition (Blue Cheese Dip): Fat: 16 g; Protein: 2.78 g; Carbs: 2.4 g; Fiber: 0.2 g; Calories: 155

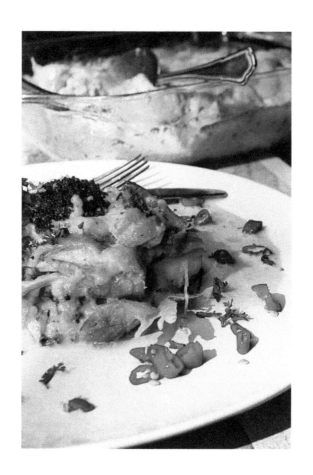

5 Tacos

Preparation Time: 10 minutes

Cooking Time: 25 minutes

Servings: 2

Ingredients:

Taco shells (makes 2 taco shells)

120 g shredded cheddar cheese

Chicken:

Grilled Chicken Breast Page

Filling:

½ cup mashed avocado

½ cup chopped tomatoes

¼ cup chopped onions

¼ cup sour cream

Parsley to garnish (optional)

Salt and pepper to taste

Directions:

Taco Shells:

Preheat the oven to 375°F (190°C)

Line a pan with parchment paper. I like to trace 2.5-inch circles on each parchment.

Measure 30 g of shredded cheese per circle and spread evenly.

Bake for 5 minutes or until little holes have appeared on the surface, and the edges begin to brown.

Remove from the oven and let cool for just a second. Remove to wooden spoons or spatulas suspended by glasses to shape taco shells.

Cool completely.

Chicken:

Cut the chicken into small pieces.

Take the tacos and add the fillings –first the chicken, then the avocado, tomatoes, onions, and sour cream. Garnish with some fresh herb such as parsley.

Season with salt and pepper to taste.

Quick Tip: While you are busy making these tacos, make a few extra because they freeze quite well and will save you some time when you make a taco dish again.

Nutrition: Fat: 63 g; Protein: 76 g; Carbs: 11.5 g; Fiber: 5 g; Calories: 918

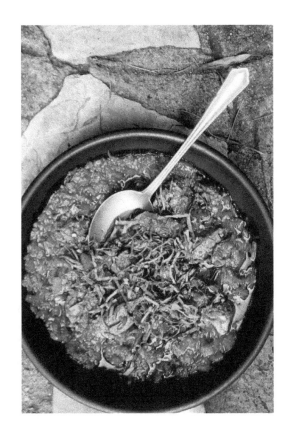

6 Chicken Livers

Preparation Time: 10 minutes

Cooking Time: 25 minutes

Servings: 2

Ingredients:

250 g chicken livers

4tbsp butter

½ large onion finely chopped

3 cloves of garlic, crushed

2 red chilies, finely chopped (optional)

½ cup white wine

1 tbsp tomato paste

1 tbsp lemon juice

1 tbsp olive oil

Salt and pepper

½ cup basil, finely chopped

Directions:

For the sauce

Place a medium-size frying pan on medium heat. Add 2 tablespoons of butter and the onion. Sauté until soft. Now add the garlic and chili. Sauté until fragrant.

Add the wine and reduce by half. Add the tomato paste and lemon juice, and let it simmer for one minute. Set aside.

Take a heavy-based frying pan and add remaining butter and olive oil. Add the chicken livers and fry them till they are beautiful and brown on both sides.

Add the sauce to the chicken livers and let it simmer until the livers are cooked.

Season to taste with salt and pepper. Now garnish with the fresh basil, and you are ready to serve.

Quick Tip: To clean your chicken livers, place the livers in cold water and let them soak for 15 minutes. This gives the water time to clot the blood, which will make it easier to remove. Drain the water and pat the livers dry with a paper towel. Look for connective tissue and trim it from the meat. Chop the liver in even, bite-size pieces.

Nutrition: Fat: 36 g; Protein: 22.6g; Carbs: 7.8 g; Fiber: 1.2 g; Calories: 489

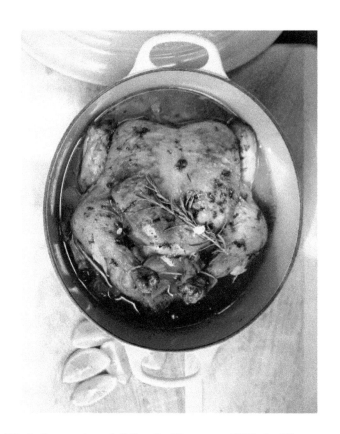

7 Chicken And Herb Butter With Keto Zucchini Roll-Ups

Preparation Time: 15 minutes

Cooking Time: 40 minutes

Servings: 4

Ingredients:

zucchini roll-ups:

1½ lb (680 g) zucchini

½ tsp salt

3 oz (85 g) butter

6 oz (170 g) mushrooms, finely chopped

6 oz (170 g) cream cheese

6 oz (170 g) shredded cheddar cheese

½ green bell pepper, chopped

2 oz (57 g) air-dried chorizo, chopped

1 egg

1 tsp onion powder

2 tbsp fresh parsley, chopped

½ tsp salt

¼ tsp pepper

Chicken:

4 (6-oz / 170-g) chicken breasts

Salt and freshly ground pepper, to taste

1 oz (28 g) butter, for frying

Herb butter:

4 oz (113 g) butter, at room temperature

1 garlic clove

½ tsp garlic powder

1 tbsp fresh parsley, finely chopped

1 tsp lemon juice

½ tsp salt

Directions:

Preheat the oven to 350°F (180°C). Cut the zucchini lengthwise into equal slices, half an inch thick. Pat dry with paper towels or a clean kitchen towel, and place on a baking tray lined with parchment paper. Sprinkle salt on the zucchini and let stand for 10 minutes.

Bake for 20 minutes in the oven, or until the zucchini is tender. Transfer to a cooling rack from the oven. Dry more if needed.

Put the butter in the saucepan over medium heat. Cut the mushrooms; put them in and stir fry well. Let cool.

Add the remaining ingredients for the zucchini roll-ups to a bowl except a third of the shredded cheese. Add the mushrooms and blend well.

Place a large amount of cheese on top of each zucchini slice. Roll up and put inside the baking dish with seams down; sprinkle on top the remainder of the cheese.

Raise the temperature to 400°F (205°C). Bake for 20 minutes, or until the cheese turns bubbly and golden.

In the meantime, season your chicken and fry it over medium heat in butter until it is crispy outside and well cooked.

Herb butter:

To prepare the herb butter, mix the butter, garlic, garlic powder, fresh parsley, lemon juice, and salt thoroughly in a small bowl. Let sit for 30 minutes and serve on top of the chicken and zucchini roll-ups.

Nutrition: Calories: 913; Fat: 84 g; Carbs: 10 g; Fiber: 3g; Protein: 30 g

8 Keto Buffalo Drumsticks With Chili Aioli And Garlic

Preparation time: 10 minutes

Cooking time: 40 minutes

Servings: 4

Ingredients:

2 lb (907 g) chicken drumsticks or chicken wings

⅓ cup mayonnaise, keto-friendly

1 tbsp smoked paprika powder or smoked chili powder

1 garlic clove, minced

2 tbsp olive oil, and more for greasing the baking dish

2 tbsp white wine vinegar

1 tsp salt

1 tsp paprika powder

1 tbsp Tabasco

Directions:

Preheat the oven to 450°F (235°C).

Make the chili aioli: Combine the mayonnaise, smoked paprika powder, garlic clove, olive oil white wine vinegar, salt, paprika powder, and Tabasco for the marinade in a small bowl.

Put the drumsticks in a plastic bag, and pour the chili aioli into the plastic bag. Shake the bag thoroughly and let marinate for 10 minutes at room temperature.

Coat a baking dish with olive oil. Place the drumsticks in the baking dish and let bake in the preheated oven for 30 to 40 minutes or until they are done and have turned a nice color. Remove the chicken wings from the oven and serve warm.

Nutrition: Calories: 570; Fat: 39 g; Carbs: 3 g; Fiber: 1 g; Protein: 43 g

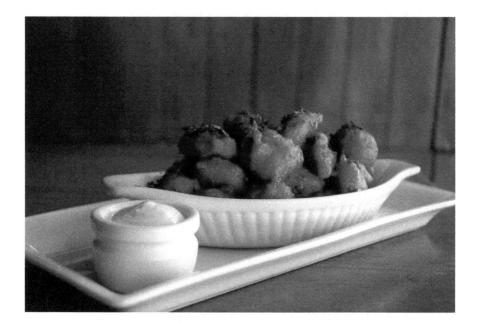

9 Mustard-Thyme Chicken with Mushrooms

Preparation Time: 10 minutes

Cooking Time: 30 minutes

Servings: 4

Ingredients:

4 chicken thighs and 4 drumsticks

2 tbsp butter

2 tbsp olive oil

1 lb (450g) sliced brown or button mushrooms

½ finely chopped onion

1 minced garlic clove

1 cup white wine

½ cup chicken stock

1 tbsp chopped fresh thyme

1 tbsp Dijon mustard

½ cup heavy cream

½ cup grated parmesan cheese

Salt and pepper to taste

Directions:

Take a large pan and melt the butter and olive oil over medium-high heat.

Place the chicken in the pan and brown on both sides, about 4 minutes on each side. Remove the chicken from the pan and set aside.

Add sliced mushrooms, onion, and garlic to the pan. Sauté for a few minutes until mushrooms are slightly limp.

Add the white wine, chicken stock, and thyme, scraping up all the bits in the bottom of the pan.

Add chicken back to pan and simmer, uncovered, for about 15-20 minutes.

Stir in the Dijon mustard, cream, and parmesan cheese. When the cheese has melted, and the sauce has come together, season to taste with salt and pepper.

Quick Tip: Dijon mustard makes so many dishes so delicious; even King Louis XI didn't travel without mustard. Peppercorns are the most used spice in the United States, and mustard comes in second. So, here's a quick tip: Dijon mustard works as an emulsifier in vinaigrette, meaning it helps the oil blend into vinegar without separating.

Nutrition: Fat: 39 g; Protein: 36 g; Carbs: 8 g; Fiber: 2 g; Calories: 520

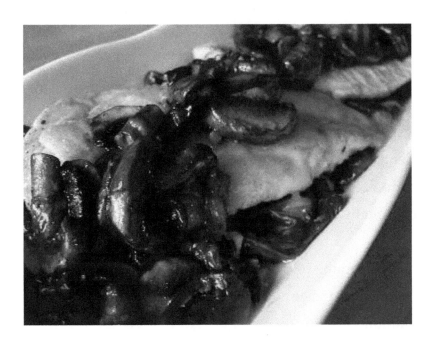

10 Chicken Francese

Preparation Time: 10 minutes

Cooking Time: 25 minutes

Servings: 2

Ingredients:

2 medium-sized boneless and skinless chicken breasts, cut in half horizontally to make 4 fillets

2 eggs

1/4 cup finely grated parmesan cheese

2 tbsp fresh lemon juice

¼ cup almond flour

2 tbsp butter

4 tbsp olive oil

4 crushed garlic cloves

½ cup dry white wine

1 cup chicken stock

¼ cup fresh parsley chopped

1 cup heavy cream

Salt and pepper to taste

Directions:

Start with the sauce. While it is reducing, you can start with the chicken.

For the sauce:

Take a medium-sized pan on medium heat and add 1 tablespoon olive oil. Add the crushed garlic, and cook until fragrant. Add in the white wine, chicken stock, and parsley. Let it reduce to about a third, stirring occasionally. Reduce the heat and add the cream. Simmer on low heat until slightly thickened.

Add salt and pepper to taste to the sauce.

For the chicken:

If the chicken breasts are not even in thickness, flatten them with a meat hammer.

In a medium-sized bowl, whisk together eggs, parmesan cheese, lemon juice, salt, and black pepper.

Place the almond flour in a shallow bowl.

Add butter and 3 tablespoons olive oil into a medium-sized pan and put it over medium to hot heat. Place one chicken fillet in the almond flour flip over to coat both sides. Then place the chicken in the egg mixture and coat it thoroughly. Place the chicken in the heated pan and fry for about 4 minutes on each side until golden brown, or until it is cooked through.

Pace the chicken on a plate and drizzle over the sauce. Garnish with a dash of parsley.

Quick Tip: If you do not like almond flour, you can substitute it with coconut flour.

Nutrition: Fat: 99 g; Protein: 75 g; Carbs: 12 g; Fiber: 1.5 g; Calories: 1292

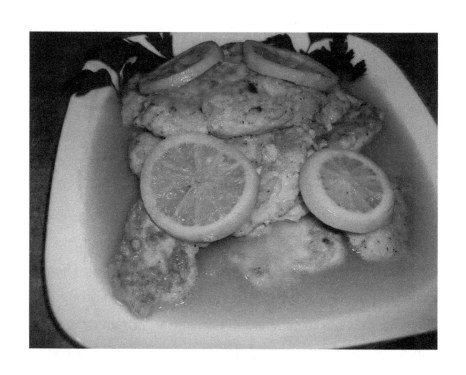

CPSIA information can be obtained
at www.ICGtesting.com
Printed in the USA
BVHW061410250221
601119BV00001B/170